HLRCC
Family Alliance
knowledge saves

WELCOME FRIEND

Chances are that if you are reading this page, you or someone you know has been impacted by HLRCC. We are very glad that you are here; to gather information, learn about this condition, and most importantly, to take control of your own, your patient's, or your loved one's health.

If you want a quick overview of HLRCC, there is a summary called "QUICK FACTS" in this book to keep handy. A printable version is included on the website.

The term HLRCC did not exist a few years ago. Previously, this disorder was thought to be two separate conditions , known as Reed's syndrome or alternately, as "MCUL". In 2001, clinical researchers linked several benign aspects of the disorder to the possibility of developing kidney cancer. At the same time, others discovered that changes to the FH gene were responsible for all of the disorder's symptoms — giving rise to the new term HLRCC. Communicating to the outside world about this condition has been slow and arduous, although we are making progress. So far, up to 1000 individuals have been involved in studies regarding this condition, but most likely thousands more individuals are going undiagnosed. In our attempt to protect ourselves and our family members, those of us diagnosed with HLRCC have learned the value of annual screening. If people with HLRCC are going to stay healthy, they have to understand the risks and take action to protect themselves. These facts, along with the knowledge that most doctors do not even know that this condition exists, prompted us to create this handbook.

The purpose of the HLRCC Family Alliance Handbook is:

To teach patients how to take control of their own health once they are diagnosed

To provide medical professionals with a convenient summary of the latest information available on HLRCC, and how best to manage the health of a patient with HLRCC.

To communicate the importance of both screening for kidney tumors and conducting genetic testing for blood-related family members

To offer doctors and patients resources for clinical research, tips for efficient and safe screening, and the most up-to-date information possible regarding current research and statistics for HLRCC

To support those HLRCC families who have a child with Fumarase Deficiency (fumaric aciduria).

Finally, it is our hope that the HLRCC Family Alliance through its website, Facebook group, and this Handbook will provide you with emotional

THE

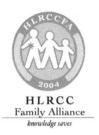

HLRCC
Family Alliance
knowledge saves

HLRCC

HANDBOOK

VERSION 2.0, MARCH 2013

Written by the HLRCC Family Alliance, a project of
the VHL Family Alliance.

Edited by Graham J. Lovitt, editor-in-chief
Assisted by:
Julie Haff Rejman
Lindsay Middelton, RN, CGC
Joyce Wilcox Graff, MA
Alison Smith

Hereditary Leiomyomatosis and Renal Cell Cancer
is a very rare genetic condition that was named
in 2001. This handbook has been created to help
educate and support all those impacted by HLRCC.

Published by Garnet Star Publishing
Boston - London - Sydney

Cover design by Susan Milliken

HLRCC Family Alliance
c/o VHL Family Alliance
2001 Beacon Street, Suite 208
Boston, MA 02135 USA
Tel/fax: + 1-617-277-5667
info@hlrccinfo.org
http://www.hlrccinfo.org

International Edition, Version 2.0
Copyright © 2012, 2013 HLRCC Family Alliance
All rights reserved

English language paperback, ISBN 978-0-9882579-7-9
English language ebook, ISBN 978-0-9882579-8-6

Library of Congress Control Number: 2013933568

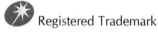 Registered Trademark

Garnet Star Publishing, Boston, Massachusetts

support. An additional online resource is Inspire (**http://vhl.inspire.com** where those impacted by HLRCC, VHL, and BHD can exchange information, stories and encouraging words. We encourage you to join and partake. They are wonderful resources!

Thank you for your support and for doing all you can to spread the word about HLRCC. Remember, KNOWLEDGE SAVES.

http://www.hlrccinfo.org

http://vhl.inspire.com

http://www.facebook.com/groups/hlrcc/

http://hlrcc.rareconnect.org

Warmly,

Julie Haff Rejman, Chair

Hereditary Leiomyomatosis and Renal Cell Cancer (HLRCC) Family Alliance

c/o VHL Family Alliance
2001 Beacon Street, Suite 208
Boston, MA 02135-7787 USA
Tel: +1 800 767-4845 ext. 709 (toll-free)
or +1 617 277-5667 ext. 709
Fax: +1 866-209-0288 (toll-free) or +1 858-712-8712
E-mail: info@hlrccinfo.org

The HLRCC Family Alliance is indebted to the
VHL Family Alliance for their generous financial
and administrative support. Although the
HLRCC syndrome is not linked to von Hippel-
Lindau (VHL), or Birt-Hogg-Dubé (BHD), they
are all related on the path to kidney cancer, and
the three syndromes have a number of common
characteristics.

See http://www.vhl.org/
and http://www.bhdsyndrome.org/

THE
HLRCC
HANDBOOK

CONTENTS

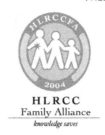

HLRCC
Family Alliance
knowledge saves

ABOUT THE
HLRCC FAMILY ALLIANCE

At the urging of Lindsay Middelton, Genetic Counselor at the US-National Cancer Institute, and with the support of Joyce Graff of the VHL Family Alliance, Phil Thayer founded the HLRCCFA in the autumn of 2004 and continued as leader of the group until early 2011.

In February 2011, Julie Haff Rejman became the Chair of the organization. Graham Lovitt became the Vice Chair. In January 2013, Antony Horton, Ph.D., also became a Vice Chair.

HLRCC Family Alliance Leadership

Chair: Julie Haff Rejman, Colorado, USA
Vice Chair: Antony Horton Ph.D., New York, USA
Vice Chair: Graham Lovitt, UK
Director of Wellness: Joyce Graff, M.A., Massachusetts, USA
VHLFA Executive Director: Ilene Sussman Ph.D.,
  Massachusetts, USA

HANDBOOK CO-EDITORS

Graham Lovitt, Editor-in-Chief
Julie Haff Rejman, Editor
Lindsay Middelton, RN, CGC
Joyce Wilcox Graff, Editor
Alison Smith, Editor

HANDBOOK CONTRIBUTORS AND REVIEWERS

Julie Adam, Ph.D.
Pamela Stratton, M.D.
Ian Tomlinson, Ph.D.

WEBSITE SUPPORT AND DESIGN:

Website designer: Angela Render
Original logo design: Dr. Daniel Rejman DDS, MS
Digital logo graphic: Ingrid Morris

Privacy Policy

The HLRCCFA website, hlrccinfo.org, subscribes to the HONcode principles of the International Health on Net Foundation, to assure you of the highest quality of health information.

Medical information on this site is reviewed by our Medical, Research and Support Council.

Information provided in this Handbook and on the website is designed to support, not replace, the relationship that exists between a patient or site visitor and his or her physician.

The website does not accept advertising. It is supported solely by donations from people with HLRCC, their friends, their families and supporters, and physicians and researchers interested in HLRCC.

We comply with the HONcode standard for trustworthy health information. Additional principles may be found in the HONcode codes of conduct, to which we adhere.

Privacy

Personal details that you provide to the HLRCC Family Alliance, including e-mail addresses, are kept entirely confidential. These details are shared within this organization among staff and volunteers for the purpose of providing service to you, but are never shared with, rented or sold to other organizations. All staff and volunteers have made confidentiality agreements to protect your information. To verify your information or send corrections, please contact us. http://www.hlrccinfo.org, Contact Us.

Information you submit to us voluntarily through the website is stored on our secure server using SSL encryption technology.

Computer Tracking and Cookies

The website is not set up to track, collect or distribute personal information not entered by visitors. Our site logs do generate certain kinds of non-identifying site usage data, such as the number of hits and visits to our sites. This information is used for internal purposes by technical support staff to provide better services to the public and may also be provided to others, but again, the statistics contain no personal information and cannot be used to gather such information.

The website also recognizes the online site where a visitor searched to find a subject which brought them to the VHL website, but we cannot identify the visitor or the visitor's address. Site information is used to help us serve these search sites with the correct information about our material, No personal information is collected.

A cookie is a small amount of data that is sent to your browser from a Web server and stored on your computer's hard drive. HLRCCFA does not use cookies in its web pages. We do not generate personal data, do not read personal data from your machine and do not store any information other than what you voluntarily submit to us.

Problems or Complaints with HLRCCFA Privacy Policy

If you have a complaint about HLRCCFA compliance with this privacy policy, you may contact us at info@hlrccinfo.org.

Links to Third Party Sites

The links included within the service may let you leave this site. The linked sites are not under the control of HLRCC Family Alliance and HLRCCFA is not responsible for the contents of any linked site, or any link contained in a linked site, or any changes or updates to such sites. These links are provided as a convenience only, and the inclusion of any link does not imply endorsement by HLRCCFA of the site or any association with their operators.

If you have technical questions about this site,

please contact info@hlrccinfo.org

Disclaimer

The content of the website should not be taken nor relied upon as medical advice on how to treat your specific manifestation of this condition. Rather, by providing context and understanding, we hope that the information provided in this Handbook and on the website will empower the patient to be a better partner in his or her own care and will facilitate constructive conversations between patient and physician. This information is intended to add to, not replace, conversations between a patient and a physician, as the specific details and the patient's total health situation need to be considered in making the final decisions about treatment.

The HLRCC Family Alliance has added a translation feature developed by Google™ Translate to assist website visitors in understanding information on this website in a variety of foreign languages. Its automated translations are not always accurate. Anyone relying on information obtained from Google™ Translate does so at his or her own risk. The HLRCCFA disclaims and will not accept any liability for damages or losses of any kind caused by the use of the Google™ Translate feature.

Medical, Research and Support Council

Links to each member can be found at
http://hlrccinfo.org/council

Julie Adam, Ph.D., Researcher, Nuffield
Department of Medicine, Oxford, UK

Kristiina Aittomäki, M.D., Ph.D., Professor,
Head of the Department of Clinical Genetics,
HUSLAB, Helsinki University Hospital,
Finland

Gennady Bratslavsky, M.D., Chair of Urology,
Upstate Medical Center, Syracuse, NY, USA

Patrick R. Carrington, M.D., Dermatologist
and Associate Editor of the Journal
of the American Academy of
Dermatology, Greenwood Village, CO, USA.

Carlos Alberto Fredes, Executive Director of the
Argentina Association of Families of Von
Hippel-Lindau (VHL-AAF) Argentina

Eyal Gottlieb, BSc., MSc., Ph.D., Research Group
Leader, Beatson Institute of Cancer Research,
Glasgow, Scotland, UK

Joyce Wilcox Graff, M.A., Director of Wellness,
VHL Family Alliance, Massachusetts, USA

Antony Horton, Ph.D., Vice Chair HLRCC
Family Alliance, previously Chief Scientific
Officer at the International Rett Syndrome
Foundation, founder and C.E.O. of his own
small company PharCited, which provides

strategic advice to the biomedical non-profit sector, New York, USA

W. Marston Linehan, M.D., Chief, Urologic Oncology Branch, National Cancer Institute*, USA

Graham Lovitt, Vice Chair HLRCC Family Alliance, retired software quality assurance manager, software systems designer, Torquay, Devon, UK

Eamonn Maher, Professor of Medical Genetics and Academic Lead for the Centre for Rare Diseases and Personalised Medicine, University of Birmingham, UK

Fred H. Menko, M.D., Ph.D., Consultant Clinical Geneticist, VU University, Amsterdam, The Netherlands

Lindsay Middelton, Genetic Counselor, National Cancer Institute*, USA

James W. Mier, M.D., Associate Professor, Department of Medicine, Harvard Medical School, USA

Patrick J Pollard, Ph.D., Beit Memorial Fellow, Nuffield Department of Medicine, Oxford, UK

Julie H. Rejman, MSW, Chair of HLRCC Family Alliance, Castle Rock, CO, USA

Stéphane Richard, M.D., Ph.D., Professor of Oncogenetics and Chair, National Expert Centre for Rare Cancers PREDIR, Le Kremlin-Bicêtre, France

Laura S. Schmidt, Ph.D., Urologic Oncology Branch, National Cancer Institute*, USA

Pamela Stratton, M.D., Gynecologist, National Institute of Child Health and Human Development, US-NIH,Bethesda, MD, USA

Sunil Sudarshan, M.D., Assistant Professor UTHSCSA, Urology, San Antonio, TX, USA

Ilene Sussman, PhD, Executive Director VHL Family Alliance, Massachusetts, USA

Min-Han Tan, MBBS, MRCP, Ph.D., Team Leader and Principal Research Scientist, Institute of Bioengineering and Nanotechnology Visiting Consultant, Medical Oncology and Cancer Genetics, National Cancer Centre Singapore

Ian Tomlinson, BA MA Ph.D. Camb, BM Brist, BM BCh Oxf, Professor of Molecular and Population Genetics, Nuffield Department of Medicine Oxford, UK

Jorge R. Toro, M.D., Investigator, Dermatology Branch, National Cancer Institute*, USA

Ingrid Winship, MB ChB, MD, FRACP, FACD., Professor of Adult Clinical Genetics, University of Melbourne and Royal Melbourne Hospital, Melbourne, Australia

*The National Cancer Institute (US-NCI) is one of the National Institutes of Health (US-NIH), Bethesda, MD, USA

Honorary Members

Although no longer actively involved, in recognition of their contribution to the world of HLRCC the following have kindly agreed to be listed as honorary members.

Virpi Launonen, Finland, Author of the paper establishing the connection between symptoms of HLRCC and the gene on chromosome 1 (2001)

Phil Thayer, USA, Founder of HLRCC Family Alliance in 2004

Supporting the HLRCC Family Alliance

The HLRCC Family Alliance was founded in 2004 as a support group for people affected by Hereditary Leiomyomatosis and Renal Cell Cancer and interested health care professionals, and to promote research. Funding the Alliance helps support our website and any outreach we do to the medical community, including such things as domestic and international mailings, attending medical conferences related to HLRCC, or supporting travel expenses for HLRCC educators.

The Alliance is funded by the generosity of its supporters. The HLRCC Family Alliance is currently not a separate legal entity and is kindly supported by VHL Family Alliance infrastructure.

* The VHL Family Alliance is registered as a non-profit charity with the tax authorities in the United States, Canada, and Great Britain, as well as other countries. Please contact your local group and your tax advisor for specific information on guidelines for tax deductibility of donations.

Please mail the following Supporter/Donation form to

HLRCC Family Alliance c/o VHLFA,
2001 Beacon Street, Suite 208,
Boston, MA 02135 USA.

Thank you!

Supporter/Donation Form

□ Yes, I want to support the HLRCC Family Alliance
c/o VHLFA
[OR]
□ I just want to make an anonymous donation

Name: _____

Address: _____

City: _____

State/Province: _____ Zip/Postcode: _____

Country (if outside the U.S.): _____

Phone daytime: _____

Phone at evening: _____

E-mail: _____

* Note all payments are tax-deductible
My check or credit card payment includes

$30 supporter*   _____

$100 contributing supporter*   _____

$250 sustaining supporter*   _____

$1000 HLRCC Research*   _____

Additional contribution*   _____

        TOTAL   _____

Payment Method:

☐ Enclosed check, payable to the VHL Family Alliance (marked for HLRCCFA)

☐ Please charge my credit card as follows:

Master Card / Visa / American Express

Card # _____

Expiration date: _____

Name as it appears on the card:

_____

Signature _____

I am a

☐ HLRCC patient

☐ HLRCC family member

☐ Supporting friend

☐ Health care professional,

Specialty : _____

☐ Other (Specify) : _____

How did you learn about the HLRCC Family Alliance?

Please list the topics you would like to see addressed on our online discussions: hlrccinfo.org, Inspire, Facebook, or RareConnect.

Your input regarding our Handbook is also welcome. Add paper as needed.

Thank you!

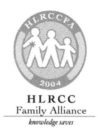

HLRCC
Family Alliance
knowledge saves

HLRCC QUICK FACTS

1. HLRCC stands for Hereditary Leiomyomatosis and Renal Cell Cancer (sometimes Carcinoma). It is also known as Reed's Syndrome.

2. HLRCC is caused by an inherited genetic alteration in the Fumarate Hydratase (FH) gene. There is a 50% risk of passing this on and the severity of the disease can vary a lot from person to person. It can be diagnosed by the detection of this genetic alteration (mutation).

3. Many women with HLRCC develop large uterine fibroids in their twenties. Although benign, the fibroids may result in early treatment.

4. Both men and women tend to develop benign skin leiomyomas (or "skin bumps") in their twenties. These two symptoms together, fibroids and skin leiomyomas, offer an important clue to the need for genetic testing of the FH gene. Because of the absence of uterine fibroids, HLRCC is more likely to go undetected in men, and early diagnosis is less likely.

5. Screening requires an annual MRI (1-3 mm slices) for the detection of kidney cancer. Be

sure to read the Handbook section "Suggested Screening Guidelines" for more information.

6. The reason why screening for HLRCC is so important is because even small HLRCC kidney tumors can metastasize, or spread, very quickly to the bones, lungs and brain. Unlike some other cancers, there is no curative treatment for kidney cancer once it metastasizes, although life may be extended with the latest class of drugs. Our goal is to prevent metastasis and stay healthy.

7. If you live in the United States, you may want to consider being part of a clinical trial at the National Institutes of Health (US-NIH) in Bethesda, MD. This is the only trial open at the time of writing. We expect that more will be opened in the future, possibly at other locations around the world.

8. It is recommended by the US-NIH that children who have a parent with HLRCC have genetic testing by age 5. There are controversies over how to screen children so please read more about this in the Handbook.

9. It is a newly identified condition (2001) and is currently being studied at several locations around the world.

10. There are approximately 200-300 families currently diagnosed with HLRCC with perhaps 1500 patients. It is an under-diagnosed condition because of its rarity.

11. Being diagnosed with HLRCC can be a very scary thing, mostly because it has the word cancer in its heading. If you have HLRCC it does

not mean that you have kidney cancer or will necessarily get it. However it does mean that you have an increased risk factor for kidney cancer, and you need to be screened so that doctors can detect even the smallest HLRCC cancer in your kidneys.

12. Our motto is *Knowledge Saves.* Although it is sometimes difficult to come to terms with a new diagnosis, we provide you and your family with information to protect yourselves and future generations. Knowledge truly is a gift.

13. We encourage you to look through our website and the Handbook. We also encourage you to reach out to us and ask for support – or offer it to another member. We are a small group, but we are very active, even on Facebook! We hope you will join us!

http://www.hlrccinfo.org

http://vhl.inspire.com

http://www.facebook/com/groups/hlrcc

http://hlrcc.rareconnect.org

The HLRCC Family Alliance
1-800-767-4845, ext 709 or +1-617-277-5667 x 709
HLRCC Family Alliance
c/o VHL Family Alliance
2001 Beacon Street, Suite 208
Boston, MA 02135-7787 USA

Enjoy this beautiful day!

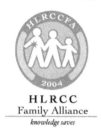

HLRCC
Family Alliance
knowledge saves

AN OVERVIEW:
WHAT IS **HLRCC**?

In recent years, scientists have used the work of the Genome Project to help identify new connections between physical symptoms that used to be viewed as isolated or random. One of these diseases is called HLRCC, or Hereditary Leiomyomatosis and Renal Cell Cancer. HLRCC is a rare inherited condition first fully described in 2001. It is caused by a tiny alteration in one copy of the FH gene.

According to researchers at the US-NIH HLRCC is a rare inherited condition characterized by the presence of cutaneous leiomyomas, uterine fibroids, and/or kidney cancer. A person who is diagnosed with HLRCC has inherited a *susceptibility* to develop one or more of these symptoms.

Approximately 450 people have been evaluated at the US-NIH, along with many other people in England, France, Japan, Finland, and Australia, but it is believed that there are many more people who are undiagnosed. Considering HLRCC is a relatively new and rare condition, there remains much to be learned.

There is considerable variation in symptoms from family to family and among members of the same family. Each person in a family has their own individual susceptibility to the symptoms. For example, if your parent had kidney cancer, it does not mean you will develop a kidney tumor. You have your own unique susceptibility.

Even if a child inherits the altered gene, it does not necessarily mean that he or she will have any symptoms of HLRCC. There may never be any symptoms at all. Or that person may develop just one of the issues, or two, or possibly all three. So far, researchers have not been able to find any patterns that would allow one to predict which symptoms a person will develop based on the particular *genotype* they have. However, there do seem to be trends in some families. Some families seem to only get leiomyomatosis and other families are more likely to get RCC (kidney cancer).

HLRCC is caused by having an alteration (mutation) in one copy of the fumarate hydratase (FH) gene. The FH gene is a section of DNA that codes for a protein called fumarase. Fumarase is an important enzyme needed for the production of energy by mitochondria, which are the tiny organelles inside our cells that produce most of our cells' energy. All people have fumarase and researchers are trying to learn the normal function of fumarase and why alterations in the FH gene cause the symptoms of HLRCC.

HLRCC is inherited in an Autosomal Dominant manner, meaning that both males and females can be affected, and each child of an affected parent has a 50% chance of inheriting the altered FH gene.

All people have two copies of the fumarate hydratase gene, one from their mother and one from their father. In a person with the condition called HLRCC, one of their two genes is normal and working well. The other is altered, meaning that it has a change in it and does not work very well. The altered FH gene is unable to produce the fumarase enzyme properly. When a person has only one working copy of the gene, their cells make less fumarase than normal, but enough to be healthy. During a person's lifetime, genes can become damaged when alterations occur during cell division or from exposure to chemicals or radiation. Cells have the ability to repair damaged DNA, but sometimes they cannot, leaving a non-working altered gene in a cell. In a person with HLRCC, an alteration in the second copy of the FH gene can lead to biochemical changes that cause those cells to grow into benign smooth muscle tumors (leiomyomas) of the skin and uterus, or less often malignant tumors of the kidney. *For more detailed information regarding the FH enzyme, please refer to our HLRCC Science document (http://www.hlrccinfo.org/science).*

Diagnostic Criteria

Although there is no consensus on diagnostic criteria, the US-NIH and other experts believe that an individual has HLRCC if they have any of the major features of the condition, including:

- Cutaneous leiomyomas: Most individuals with HLRCC present with multiple cutaneous leiomyomas (skin bumps).

- Uterine Leiomyomas: Most females with HLRCC have uterine fibroids, often quite large and occurring early in their 20s. However, fibroids are very common in the general population and are rarely diagnostically useful on their own.

- Kidney (Renal) tumors: Most people who have HLRCC **do not** develop kidney tumors. The incidence of kidney tumors in the US-NIH study group is about 30%. However, the incidence of kidney tumors in the European group is reported as much lower. We are still learning the specific factors that increase or decrease one's risk of kidney cancer.

- A positive genetic test for HLRCC: This means that an alteration has been detected in the Fumarate Hydratase gene. FH alterations can be found in about 97% of families who are strongly suspected of having HLRCC.

If HLRCC is suspected, but the genetic alteration cannot be found and there are no cutaneous leiomyomas, then a fumarase enzyme assay can be done on cells derived from skin or blood. A fumarase activity level less than or equal to 60% is indicative of HLRCC. This test is specialized and it is not available in most laboratories. Some laboratories that can test for fumarase activity find difficulties because of problems in calculating and interpreting the results.

There are other cancers which have been occasionally associated with HLRCC. Breast and prostate are examples. Some HLRCC family members have other health problems (an example is thyroid nodules), but it is not clear if these are related to HLRCC. At this point they are assumed to be coincidental. We are all still members of the general population.

Note: Researchers in England have discovered a chemical compound that is present in HLRCC tumors, but not in non HLRCC tumors (kidney and other tumors), so in the future we may see newer and better screening tests for HLRCC.

Note: There are other tumor types where the number of cases is too small to allow us to categorize these tumors as diagnostic criteria for HLRCC, but when they occur in an HLRCC patient, the tumors are found to have no fumarase activity. Examples are benign adrenal tumors and Leydig testicular cancer which develops in the Leydig cells -- the cells in the testes that release the male hormone, testosterone. There is also a possibility of benign ovarian cystadenomas being associated with HLRCC.

Genetic Testing

HLRCC is an autosomal dominant disorder. "Autosomal" means that the alteration is located on one of the 22 regular chromosomes and not on a sex chromosome (X or Y). "Dominant" means that having just one copy of the altered gene is enough to cause the disorder. *This means that if a person has HLRCC, there is a 50% chance that he or she will pass the altered gene to a child.* There is a 50% chance that an embryo of an HLRCC parent will have the condition, depending on whether the particular egg or sperm from which that the embryo was formed contained the altered copy of the gene. You have two FH genes – one from each parent. The one healthy parent gives you one healthy unaltered FH gene. The other parent with the altered gene gives you one of their two copies of the gene: either a healthy unaltered FH gene or an altered FH gene – hence the 50% chance. You either have an altered gene or you don't. Occasionally a person with an altered FH gene may have very few symptoms, so that it may seem to skip a generation, but if you do not have an altered FH gene you cannot pass it to a child. It is possible for an alteration in the FH gene to be present for the first time in one family member as a result of a mutation in a germ cell (egg or sperm) of one of the parents or in the fertilized egg itself. This is termed a "de novo mutation".

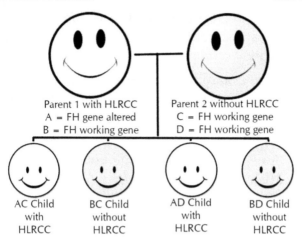

Figure 1: Inheritance of HLRCC. For more information see
http://www.nlm.nih.gov/medlineplus/ency/article/002049.htm

Each child gets one copy of the FH gene from each parent.

In this way, there are four possible arrangements of these four genes. Each arrangement has a 25% chance. So for each child there is a 50% chance of having HLRCC and a 50% chance of not having it.

Genetic testing is the most reliable way of diagnosing HLRCC. Although a physician can often diagnose an individual with HLRCC based on the physical signs listed above, the US-NIH recommend that individuals obtain genetic testing to confirm that they actually have the gene alteration.

Benefits of genetic testing to confirm HLRCC:

- A positive test (meaning you do have HLRCC) will help people advocate with

their doctors and insurance companies
for agreement with their need for annual
kidney screening.

- It gives family members who do not have
symptoms the ability to discover whether
they have the gene alteration by a simple
blood test.

- A negative test (meaning you do not have
HLRCC) can put your own fears to rest
when other family members have tested
positive (meaning they have HLRCC).

- As we learn more, the exact alteration
in your gene will become increasingly
important to your own health maintenance.

Things to keep in mind regarding genetic
testing:

- It may complicate your ability to obtain
life or health insurance. Refer to section
about Life and Health insurance. Genetic
testing and lifetime kidney surveillance is
expensive. It is much easier if a person has
health insurance in place before obtaining a
DNA test.

- It can be an emotional process. It is not
a simple blood test. The results may
be difficult to interpret, and it is best
to undertake genetic testing through a
genetic professional (geneticist or genetic
counselor) who can help you understand
the results and their implications for
yourself and your family.

- If you have your children tested before their age of consent and they are found positive there are implications for future life or health insurance, and mortgage applications as well as the start of a life-long screening process. This is a difficult decision to make between health safety and financial implications. We recommend that people have life insurance in place even for children before obtaining a DNA test. Many countries are passing anti-discrimination laws to protect citizens.

If you are in the worldwide HLRCC clinical study at the US-NIH (Bethesda, Maryland, USA):

Genetic testing at US-NIH is optional, so you can still be in the study and not have the genetic testing done. This is especially beneficial if you have physical signs and family members who have had positive genetic testing, but don't want the testing done yourself. All testing at US-NIH is optional.

If you are not in the US-NIH study, you should look for a genetic counselor from your area online. The best links to use are:

US— http://www.nsgc.org/

World— http://geneclinics.org and go to the link for Clinic Directory

You will want to bring a copy of a clinical paper about HLRCC (such as the Toro article http://www.ncbi.nlm.nih.gov/books/NBK1252/)

with you to your genetic counselor, and your genetic counselor is welcome to contact Lindsay Middelton at US-NIH or another expert consultant to obtain further information. You should also give your genetic counselor the link www. hlrccinfo.org so that they can make sure you get the screening you need when they connect you with the proper physicians, should your test be positive.

References:

- Pithukpakorn M, Toro JR, Hereditary Leiomyomatosis and Renal Cell Cancer. GeneReviews [Internet]. 2010. PMID: 20301430

- or http://www.ncbi.nlm.nih.gov/ books/NBK1252/

The risk of developing the features of HLRCC increases with age. You are at significant risk of being diagnosed with an FH gene alteration if you have a diagnosed blood relative. The actual risk figure depends on the closeness of the relationship starting as high as 50% with a first degree relative (parent, child or sibling). There is a lower risk of 25% with a second degree relative (uncle/aunt, niece/nephew or a grandparent) and a still lower risk with a third degree relative (first cousin) or even a first cousin's child. The alteration cannot however skip generations so the more genetic testing a family has the more precise the risk figure will be for each individual ranging from 0% to 50%. In other words, if one of your parents is at risk, but tests negative, then you will not be at risk. If a person does not carry the altered gene, they cannot pass it to a child. You may wish to discuss this with your genetic counselor for more clarification.

If you test positive and want to inform other family members, there is at the end of the handbook, a printable Family Letter (to send to relatives of someone recently diagnosed with HLRCC). The letter should only come from the person with the HLRCC diagnosis, or the next-of-kin if the person has died, in order to respect their privacy. It is important to keep in mind that your family members may be overwhelmed when they receive this information. We tried to keep this in mind when creating our printable letter and to offer the support of the HLRCC Family Alliance as a way of supporting each and every person associated with this condition.

If your genetic test is negative, but you have symptoms of HLRCC you should check that your genetic test covered the possibility of FH deletions, in addition to bidirectional sequencing. This is usually through a technique called MLPA or multiplex ligation probe amplification. Some companies only offer sequencing.

It can sometimes take several months to obtain genetic testing results, but once one genetic alteration is identified within the family, testing of additional family members is faster and less costly. Tests in some countries are faster than others. Please consider the following PROS and CONS when considering genetic testing as well:

PROS:

- Knowing about the HLRCC genetic alteration gives you the insight to screen and protect yourself or your siblings/children or other family members, if they are tested. Knowledge is power!

- Catching HLRCC tumors early may save your life. A kidney tumor often grows with no symptoms. Periodic screening with scans will catch a tumor early, so that it can be treated.

CONS:

- A positive test result may have an impact on your own and your children's ability to get life or health insurance. You should be sure to have coverage before requesting DNA testing.

The knowledge of a condition such as this has emotional implications. People can become very worried about the future, which is where a support group such as HLRCC Family Alliance **www.hlrccinfo.org** can help to put your life back on track.

Life and Health Insurance

A useful link describing the general implications for insurance (applies to all genetic conditions not just to Birt-Hogg-Dubé) is

http://www.bhdsyndrome.org/for-families/additional-resources/insurance/

and there is information for different US States in

http://www.healthinsuranceinfo.net/ and
http://healthcare.gov

Concerns about Genetic Discrimination

Many people who learn they may have HLRCC are concerned that their health insurance company will either terminate their policy or deny coverage if the insurer learns of their genetic status.   Many states have enacted state laws to protect their citizens from genetic discrimination by health insurers.   However, the protection offered varies widely among state laws. You can access information about your state law by accessing http://genome.gov > Issues in Genetics > Statute and Legislation Database (http://www.genome.gov/PolicyEthics/LegDatabase/pubsearch.cfm)

In 2008 the Genetic Information Nondiscrimination Act (GINA) was signed into law. The GINA Act prohibits discrimination by health insurance companies and employers based on "genetic information", including information about genetic testing or your results (and those of your family members) or information about family history of any disease or disorder.

Health insurance protection:

- Group and individual health insurers may not use your genetic information to set eligibility, premium or contribution amounts;

- Health insurers may not request or require that you take a genetic test.

Employment protection:

- Employers may not use your genetic information to make decisions involving hiring, firing, job assignments and promotions;

- Employers may not request, require or purchase genetic information about you or one of your family members.

GINA stipulates that genetic information alone cannot be considered a pre-existing condition.

What does GINA NOT do?

- GINA does NOT restrict health care providers from requesting, offering or providing information about a genetic test to patients.

- GINA does NOT require insurance companies to pay for any particular test.

- GINA does NOT apply to life, disability or long term insurance.

- If you have been diagnosed with a medical problem or a symptom related to HLRCC, GINA does NOT apply.

Employers with fewer than 15 employees and the military are not required to abide by the employment protections.

Having Children

Deciding whether to have children when there is a 50% chance of inheriting a problem is a difficult decision to make. Before making any decision you may wish to speak with a geneticist or genetic counselor about possible testing options and their implications.

One option may be Pre-implantation Genetic Diagnosis (PGD). There is information on the VHL Family Alliance website about PGD. See http://www.vhl.org/?s=pgd

Other options may include Chorionic Villus Sampling (CVS) or amniocentesis.

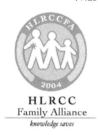

HLRCC
Family Alliance
knowledge saves

CUTANEOUS LEIOMYOMAS (SKIN BUMPS)

There is considerable variation in the appearance of cutaneous leiomyomas as can be seen in the following photographs making it difficult to diagnose by sight unless you are a specialist. See Figures 2-5.

Just as uterine leiomyomas grow from smooth muscle of the uterus, cutaneous leiomyomas are rare benign tumors that grow from smooth muscles in the skin. The arrectores pilorum (singular arrector pili, also called piloerectus muscles) are small smooth muscles that are attached to hair follicles. These are the muscles that allow your hairs to "stand up" when you are cold or fearful. When benign tumors grow from arrrectores pilorum, they are called piloleiomyomas. sometimes pilar leiomyomas and often just cutaneous leiomyomas. It is estimated that most people with HLRCC will get one or more piloleiomyomas in their lifetime. Piloleiomyomas are very helpful for identifying people who are likely to have HLRCC.

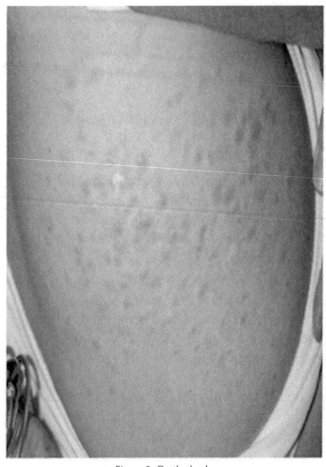

Figure 2: On the back.
Photo courtesy of Dr. Ed Cowen, NIH, NCI.

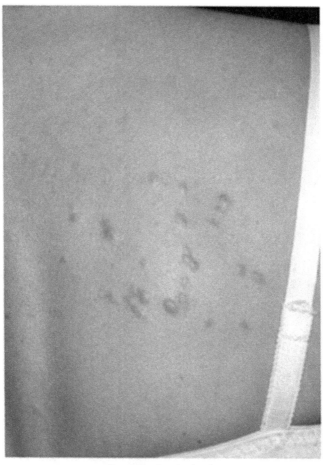

Figure 3: On the back.
Photo courtesy of Dr. Ed Cowen, NIH, NCI.

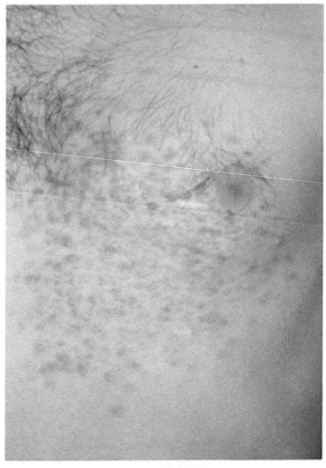

Figure 4. On the chest.
Photo courtesy of Dr. Ed Cowen, NIH, NCI.

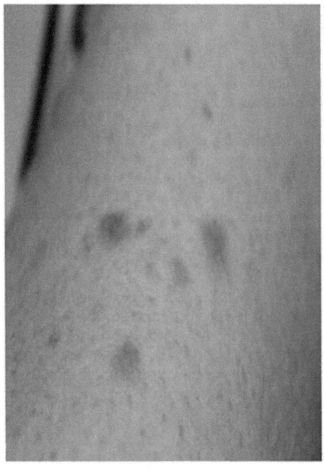

Figure 5. On the leg.
Photo courtesy of an HLRCC patient.

Individuals who have HLRCC tend to have cutaneous leiomyomas by the time they are in their 30's, but some have gotten them as early as 11 years old; some people report finding their first one in their 50's. They tend to grow anywhere on the body and limbs, but rarely on the face, hands or feet. These bumps can be very small, but sometimes large, can range in color from skin-colored to light brown to red, and tend to grow in mosaic clusters, but can also be solitary. Some people have a single leiomyoma, but many people develop small clusters of leiomyomas. A smaller percentage of people develop wide distribution of leiomyomas over a chest or back ("segmental distribution"). Once a leiomyoma appears, it does not normally go away and others may appear over the following years.

Leiomyomas can be mistaken for post-acne scarring. They are very firm to the touch and discrete as compared to acne or eczema. They are not common skin lesions in the general population, but dermatologists are starting to recognize them more easily as potential indicators of HLRCC.

Diagnosis

A skin biopsy MUST be done to confirm a leiomyoma, as relying on appearance is inconclusive. A skin biopsy involves minor surgical removal of some of the skin bump, after which the tissue is sent to a pathology lab. An anesthetic agent is injected under the skin around the leiomyoma and once the area is numb, a small sample of tissue is taken. Slides are prepared from the tissue and examined under a microscope by a pathologist to determine whether the diagnosis is piloleiomyoma or some other type of growth. Cutaneous leiomyomas can be the only clue to a physician about whether a person is at risk for HLRCC. If one has a first-degree relative with HLRCC, then a single confirmed cutaneous leiomyoma is sufficient for the diagnosis of HLRCC.

Pain

As with all the conditions associated with HLRCC there is considerable variation not only in the appearance of cutaneous leiomyomas, but also in the experience of pain in them. The exact cause of pain has not been understood, but there is a thought that the leiomyoma has trapped nerve cells. The variation is not just from patient to patient, but also within one patient and can increase over time. Some patients find a cold sensitivity to such an extent that they even consider moving to a warmer country. Some find that if a pain develops in one leiomyoma it acts as a trigger to all the others to become also painful for hours or days at a time. Sometimes a leiomyoma that grows initially without having any pain symptom can start to become irritable and painful. Pain can sometimes occur as a result of exertion, or by touch or rubbing clothes. When pain does occur most patients describe it as excruciating, like having a knifepoint stab.

Treatment

Most dermatologists do NOT recommend surgically removing all these growths, except as needed for biopsies, as it tends to cause scarring and divots in the skin where the procedure is performed. However painful or unsightly leiomyomas, if there are not too many close together, can be surgically removed using CO_2 laser or cryosurgery. Preferably the removal is by a skilled plastic surgeon to minimize scarring. Use of a super-fine thread avoids the dots on either side of the line of surgery. Removal will normally be done under a local anesthetic. There is a reported case of extensive multiple piloleiomyomas being successfully removed by surgery and reconstructed with a flap technique. Sometimes the leiomyomas will grow back after removal, possibly because some tissue was left behind, or there were new ones growing in a cluster. You should talk with a dermatologist about what is best for your type of skin growth.

Currently researchers at US-NIH are experimenting with Botox therapy to help with the pain (see Clinical Trials). If you have painful cutaneous leiomyomas, you may want to get a contact name from info@hlrccinfo.org or talk with your own dermatologist about the various options for pain control.

One of our members has found significant relief using Lyrica. As with any treatment you should first discuss and agree its suitability with your physician and or dermatologist. The links below have a lot of information about Lyrica including descriptions of warnings and side effects which seem important to study before deciding to take it.

- http://www.lyrica.com/PHN/phn-introduction.aspx and
- http://arthritis.about.com/od/Pregabalin/a/Lyrica.htm and
- http://en.wikipedia.org/wiki/Pregabalin

Another pain relief drug that is being used is niphediprine. As with the use of all drugs you should consult with your medical team—especially so if intending to become pregnant.

Significant pain relief has also been reported with pulsed hysocine butyl bromide see http://www.ncbi.nlm.nih.gov/pubmed/20049277 . This article mentions many calcium channel blockers like nifedipine, phenoxybenzamine, doxazocine, gabapentin and topical 9% hyoscine hydrobromide.

A dermatologist should conduct an annual inspection of all cutaneous leiomyomas to detect changes which might lead to malignant leiomyosarcoma (which is a rare cancer). There has been one reported case of a solitary angioleiomyoma with multiple piloleiomyomas see http://www.ncbi.nlm.nih.gov/pubmed/10356411 .

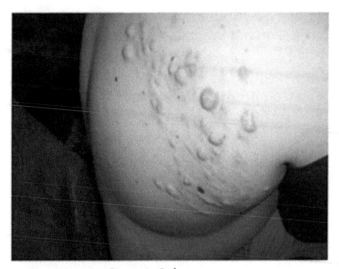

Figure 6. Before surgery

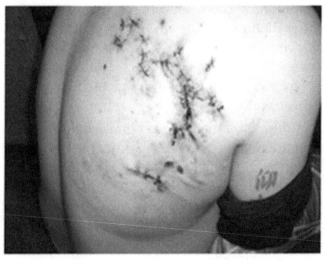

Figure 7. Three days after surgery
Photos courtesy of Ryan N.

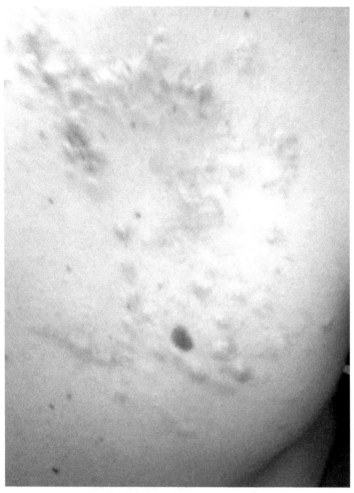

Figure 8. Healed, with some regrowth..
Photos courtesy of Ryan N.

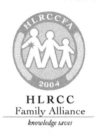

HLRCC
Family Alliance
knowledge saves

UTERINE FIBROIDS

Like the skin, the uterus contains smooth muscle tissue, and uterine fibroids are smooth muscle tumors that grow in the wall of the uterus or womb. They are almost always benign (non-cancerous) and can be as small as an apple seed or as large as a grapefruit. Another medical term for fibroids is uterine leiomyoma or just myoma.

In the general population, up to 80% of women develop uterine fibroids by the age of 50 years. Uterine fibroids are the leading reason for hysterectomies in the United States (1 in 3 have fibroids). Women with fibroids may be at greater risk of having a cesarean section when they give birth. Other women with fibroids may have difficulty becoming pregnant or carrying a pregnancy. More often fibroids are simply "innocent bystanders" during pregnancy and cause no problems at all.

Uterine fibroids are often the first physical symptom to develop in a female who has HLRCC. Although a nuisance, they provide a clue to individuals who are at risk, as well as a warning to be looking for skin leiomyomas, which are often the second physical symptoms of HLRCC.

The growth of uterine fibroids is believed to be affected by hormones (especially the female hormones estrogen and progesterone). The occurrence of fibroids is genetic. Uterine fibroids that are associated with HLRCC tend to be larger and to occur at earlier ages than in the general population.

If you are planning to have children, it may be better to have them in your 20's rather than to wait until your 30's, as over time fibroids may begin to create issues which can complicate fertility or pregnancy.

Fibroid Symptoms

Fibroids are so common — and can be so small — that many women do not even know that they have them. Women with HLRCC often have more or much larger fibroids that are accompanied by other symptoms, including:

- Heavy bleeding
- A feeling of fullness in the pelvic area
- Enlargement of the abdomen
- Frequent urination
- Pain during sex
- Lower back pain
- Complications during pregnancy and labor

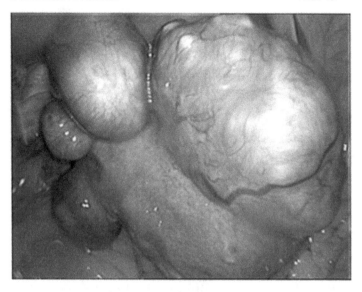

Figure 9. Fibroid tumors seen during surgery.
From http://en.wikipedia.org/wiki/Uterine_fibroid

Diagnosis

Ways to find out if you have uterine fibroids:

- A gynecology (GYN) pelvic examination (a doctor can often detect larger fibroids just by feeling the abdomen).
- An ultrasound scan
- MRI scan
- Hysterosalpingogram — where dye is injected into the uterus

A pelvic ultrasound scan is usually performed transvaginally. However, when the uterus is very large, a transabdominal pelvic ultrasound may be needed to measure the full size of the fibroids and uterus. Some radiologists and gynecologists also perform a sonohysterogram in which a catheter is placed in the cervix into the uterus and fluid (sterile water or saline) is infused. Sonohysterograms can be helpful in determining whether there are fibroids within the uterine cavity.

Hysterosalpingogram is an x-ray test done during testing for infertility, and is used to investigate the shape of the uterine cavity and the whether the fallopian tubes may be blocked. During hysterosalpingograms, radio-opaque material is injected into the uterine cavity and x-rays are done. Hysterosalpingograms can be helpful in determining whether there are fibroids within the uterine cavity or whether these fibroids compress the opening to the fallopian tubes. However they are not useful in looking at the fibroids themselves, and not all centers perform this procedure.

A gynecologist should conduct an annual examination of women to check for an increase in uterine size suggestive of fibroids. Once a woman with HLRCC is known to have fibroids, a gynecologist should continue these annual checks and consider adding radiological examination. Having imaging studies done over time (ultrasound or MRI) will also enable the radiologist and gynecologist to determine whether the fibroids have grown in size or number. Significant growth in fibroid size might suggest the development of a malignant type of fibroids called leiomyosarcoma. Thus, when fibroids grow rapidly, surgical treatment is usually recommended. Hysterosonograms and hysterosalpingograms may be helpful as a preoperative assessment for myomectomy (described below). While the first reports of HLRCC suggested that leiomyosarcoma might occur in women with fibroids, a large study at US-NIH has shown that fibroids may be atypical, but no cases of leiomyosarcoma have been observed.

> *A moving story :*
>
> "I was at the University of Michigan as a high risk patient while I was pregnant with my first child," said Julie Sherwood, a 39-year-old HLRCC patient. "I had a vertical c-section and they still could not find my baby because I had so many fibroids in the way. They had to do a second incision and the baby was saved. During my second pregnancy my fibroids tripled within weeks and the baby couldn't survive. I had an emergency hysterectomy weeks later."
>
> Julie's moving story, along with many other discussions about a variety of health-related topics, can be found in a recent radio interview at: http://www.powerfulpatient.org/?p=1006

Treatment

There are several options of managing fibroids. Many factors are considered to determine which option is the best one for each individual.

Sometimes a hysterectomy is recommended. During hysterectomy the uterus and cervix are removed, and sometimes the ovaries are removed as well. It is not possible to carry a pregnancy after the uterus is removed.

Another option for treating fibroids is a surgical procedure called myomectomy. During a myomectomy only the fibroids are removed, and thus the ability to carry a pregnancy may be preserved. When fibroids are within the uterine cavity, they may be removed through a hysteroscopic myomectomy procedure (operating using a viewing instrument through the cervix).

When the fibroids are large and within the wall of the uterus, an abdominal myomectomy is usually performed. While some gynecologists perform this procedure laparoscopically or robotically (operating using a viewing instrument in the abdomen), it is important that the fibroids are not morcellated (mechanically cut up into pieces) inside your body. Removing the fibroid intact will enable the pathologist to examine it for atypical features or possible leiomyosarcoma. Additionally, there is a concern that many fibroids associated with HLRCC are atypical and cellular. With morcellation, small pieces of tissue left in your body may attach and grow.

Another concern is the number of myomectomy procedures done prior to attempting pregnancy. If a woman undergoes several myomectomy procedures prior to attempting pregnancy, she may have difficulty becoming pregnant or may be at risk of miscarriage. These effects may occur because, for example, of scarring in the uterine wall. Thus, timing myomectomy surgery just before attempting pregnancy may be a preferable strategy.

Non-surgical treatments of uterine fibroids include Uterine Artery Embolization (UAE) or High Intensity Focused Ultrasound Ablation (HIFU) of fibroids. Both procedures are performed by an interventional radiologist. These physicians are trained in a medical sub-specialty of radiology which utilizes minimally-invasive image-guided procedures to treat diseases. At the present time, neither procedure is recommended for women with HLRCC as they will not investigate whether fibroids are atypical or cancerous. *These strategies either lessen the flow of blood to the uterus (UAE) or physically destroy part of the fibroid (HIFU).* In some patients with HLRCC who have undergone UAE, their fibroids have rapidly increased in size.

Birth control pills and the levonorgestrel (Mirena^TM) IUD decrease menstrual bleeding in women regardless of whether they have fibroids, and are effective methods of contraception. Women with the HLRCC gene defect are able to use these treatments for these indications. *While fibroids do appear to be hormone-sensitive, it is unknown at this time whether using hormones like birth control pills or the levonorgestrel IUD will be effective in decreasing fibroid size in women with HLRCC.*

There are many organizations and links that will assist in your understanding of uterine fibroids. Keep in mind that we are currently trying to educate these organizations about HLRCC and that you most likely will not find information specific to HLRCC on these websites.

The Center for Uterine Fibroids

http://www.fibroids.net

National Uterine Fibroids Foundation

Colorado Springs, Colorado

+1 (719) 633-3454

http://www.huff.org

The following links provide additional information about fibroids:

http://www.womenshealth.gov

http://www.fibroidoptions.com/

http://www.dbh.nhs.uk/Library/ Patient_Information_Leaflets/WPR24900%20 Hysterosalpingogra.pdf

http://www.sirweb.org/patients/uterine-fibroids/

http://www.everydayhealth.com/health-center/uterine-fibroids.aspx

There are additional links for fibroids to be found in the HLRCC Science document.

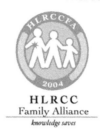

HLRCC
Family Alliance
knowledge saves

Renal (Kidney) Tumors

Research indicates that only a proportion of individuals with HLRCC develop malignant (cancerous) kidney tumors. There is a higher proportion in the US-NIH study possibly because they are recruiting as kidney cancer specialists. The variation in incidence figures is considerable and may depend on several factors including methods of recruitment. It will take more studies to determine the true risk of kidney tumors in a particular individual. Meanwhile, since this is such a potentially lethal tumor, we recommend that everyone be screened for kidney tumors. See Suggested Screening Guidelines.

Diagnosis

Kidney cancer often develops with no initial symptoms, and by the time symptoms such as pain or blood in the urine appear, it has often already become a danger to life.

In the general population kidney cancer accounts for about 3% of all cancers. Whereas the cell type of most kidney cancers is Clear

Cell, HLRCC tumors are most often called Type II Papillary, sometimes Tubulopapillary, occasionally Collecting Duct Carcinoma, and rarely Clear Cell.

Dr. Maria Merino of the US-National Cancer Institute described the typical features of the HLRCC tumors in *"The morphologic spectrum of kidney tumors in hereditary leiomyomatosis and renal cell carcinoma (HLRCC) syndrome"*:

A person with a diagnosis of HLRCC has a much higher risk of developing lesions in the kidney compared to the general population. There are three kinds of lesions in the kidney: benign cysts, hard tumors, and hard lumps developing inside a cyst.

Unlike other genetic syndromes associated with kidney cancer, HLRCC kidney tumors can metastasize (spread) when the tumor is relatively small (less than 1 cm). These tumors usually spread to the lungs, bone and brain. It was thought that HLRCC was generally unilateral in that only one kidney is initially affected. However as people are living longer after surgery, problems can develop in the remaining kidney.

Like all kidney tumors they often initially have few, if any, noticeable symptoms, which is why scanning is essential in order to detect them at an earlier stage.

Merino MJ, Torres-Cabala C, Pinto P, Linehan WM., 2007
http://www.ncbi.nlm.nih.gov/pubmed/17895761

Treatment / Management of the Kidneys

This is an area which is still being actively researched and there are many factors to be considered for every individual. The key to managing HLRCC kidney tumors is surveillance to find tumors when they are small. Surgical removal if possible is currently the treatment of choice when a tumor is found. Some families report a currently healthy grandparent who had a nephrectomy many years ago, and there are people who had tumors removed 10 years ago who are healthy and well.

Once an HLRCC kidney tumor has metastasized, the prognosis changes, and the course of metastatic kidney cancer is similar to the experience of others in the general population. There are targeted molecular treatments that are currently in clinical trials. At the US-NIH there is a clinical trial of a combination of bevacizumab (Avastin) and erlotinib (Tarceva). The spectrum of available drugs and the recommendations for primary and secondary therapies for papillary kidney cancer is evolving rapidly. Check with an oncologist experienced in kidney cancer and make contact with an HLRCC specialist with advice from info@hlrccinfo.org.

The type of kidney surgery is dependent on many factors. Sometimes it may be necessary to remove the entire kidney (nephrectomy) or a partial nephrectomy may be performed. A partial nephrectomy is nephron sparing surgery in which only the tumor and a little surrounding margin of tissue is removed.

Follow-up after RCC

The exact follow-up procedure for every patient will vary from center to center and should be discussed and agreed with your physicians. **We will only describe here examples of what you may expect.**

If you have had a nephrectomy, then initially for the first 2 years a full chest and abdominal CT scan with contrast may be carried out every 6 months to check for any metastasis (spread). **ALWAYS TELL THE RADIOLOGIST THAT YOU HAVE ONLY ONE KIDNEY AND PLEASE TO REDUCE THE AMOUNT OF CONTRAST.**

A PET/CT and a bone scan may also be ordered if metastasis is thought likely. Kidney cancer will often metastasize to the lungs or bone. Note this is then called secondary kidney cancer in the lung or bone and NOT lung cancer or bone cancer.

After two years the screening interval may be increased to yearly, but there continues to be a life-time risk of either recurrence or metastasis requiring long-term surveillance. See http://www.ncbi.nlm.nih.gov/pubmed/21903243

Types of Scans

There are four types of Kidney Imaging: Magnetic Resonance Imaging (MRI), Computed Tomography (CT), Positron Emission Tomography (PET) and Ultrasound. Some centers will alternate MRI with CT scans. The kidney cancer of HLRCC can metastasize (spread to other organs or bone) even when small, which makes early detection essential. There are several well used methods to visualize kidney tumors. There are pros and cons for each.

Magnetic Resonance Imaging (MRI)

MRI scans with and without contrast is an acceptable method to examine kidneys. This process creates images using magnetic waves. No radiation is used.

The MRI scan should use thin slices or "cuts" from 1-3 mm and this should be ordered by your physician. Radiologists resist thin cuts because they take up computer storage space and the scan is longer. The preferred option is to use MRI with gadolinium contrast, because it is the contrast medium that identifies soft tissue. MRI scanners have recently improved with "Open MRI" and shorter and wider tunnels making the experience less problematic even for people with mild claustrophobia. However there is some concern that the image quality may be reduced with some open large bore MRI scanners. The objective is to get the best possible picture quality. If you feel you need calming medication for anxiety or discomfort, a larger bore to accommodate larger body mass, or any other requests, negotiate a solution that will give the doctor the picture quality needed while addressing your concerns.

Computed Tomography (CT Scan)

CT scans with and without contrast is an acceptable method of visualizing kidneys. However, images are created through the use of radiation. Annual CT scans over a life span raises concerns about using up your lifetime maximum of radiation exposure.

The CT scan is done with a contrast agent usually containing iodine and you should drink plenty of water afterwards to flush the contrast agent out of your body. If there is any doubt about your kidney function (creatinine levels above 1.6) you may be given 500cc of saline solution first and Visipaque(*iodixanol*) or Omnipaque (*iohexol*) contrast which have lower iodine content.

Positron Emission Tomography (PET)

For ordinary RCC, PET scans are normally less effective than CT scans with contrast and have been known to give false negatives. A PET scan is often combined with a CT scan. However, with HLRCC any tumors present are glucose hungry and PET can be a useful diagnostic tool especially for detecting metastases. There can be false positives in both the adrenal glands and the uterus because of the presence of benign HLRCC related tissue. Cancer cells upregulate glucose metabolism, which is a phenomenon known as the Warburg effect. This is the basis for PET in which a glucose analog tracer FDG (2-18fluoro-2-deoxy-D-glucose), a radioactive modified hexokinase substrate, is used to differentiate between normal and tumor tissue.

Ultrasound

Ultrasound can be effective in visualizing **some** kidney tumors, but can easily miss the small tumors associated with HLRCC or does not detect some types of tumor tissue. Ultrasound is used occasionally when a tumor is present to determine the amount of fluid in the mass.

> *Note:* **Ultrasound as a screening (surveillance) method is not recommended for people with HLRCC.**

Bone Scan

A bone scan consists of taking a camera image of your body about 3 to 4 hours after giving you an injection of a radioactive isotope. This can detect any metastasis that has spread to the bones.

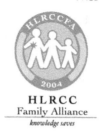

HLRCC
Family Alliance
knowledge saves

SUGGESTED SCREENING GUIDELINES

The suggestions in this book come from the most experienced research projects, which still are only 10 years old, and therefore do not yet have long-term follow-up experience. Some physicians are of the opinion that there is insufficient scientific data yet to define firm recommendations. Recommendations presented in this handbook should be regarded as tentative, and will most likely change over time as more data becomes available.

We suggest these guidelines as a starting point, and ask for feedback to help shape better guidelines in the future.

The one common guideline we do recommend is that you take charge. Be informed, discuss openly with your medical professionals and consider the pros and cons. Please e-mail us at info@hlrccinfo.org if you have unanswered questions and we will always try to help you.

HLRCC is a relatively young condition in that there are few people who have been followed medically from childhood through adulthood with today's screening technologies. We have lots of questions, but few firm answers at this time. However everyone with HLRCC can assist us in learning what we need to know to protect ourselves and our children from the worst effects of HLRCC.

The purpose of screening guidelines is to help patients and their local physicians watch out for foreshadowing of problems, before they get to a critical stage. By intervening at earlier stages, hopefully these problems never become threatening to life or quality of life. Note that *screening* means that you do not yet have any issues in the area being screened. Once you have a diagnosed issue, then you will need to follow the guidance of your health care team in deciding what course of action to take. Feel free to seek a second opinion from a doctor more familiar with HLRCC, even in another country. Scans can easily be sent through the mail, and the experts are quite willing to provide their opinion. Note: e-mailing scans is not satisfactory. There are many file formats used by the various vendors, so the receiving doctor will likely not be able to read the file. On the CD they include the viewer software to read the file, so the receiving doctor can open the file and read it quite nicely. Sending a universal format (like a .pdf) reduces the quality of the image, making it hard to determine what is a cyst and what is a tumor — a critical distinction for us.

- MRI is recommended in order to minimize exposure to radiation.
- CT should be reserved for times when they are needed to answer some

specific diagnostic question or in planning surgery.

- Ultrasound of the kidney is not recommended, as ultrasound is very much dependent upon the quality of the machine and the skill of the operator. Ultrasound is better than nothing, but is unlikely to find tumors less than 1 cm, leaving a wide opportunity for risk in HLRCC.

The screening guidelines shown in this section are the best advice we were able to assemble at this time from the major research teams studying this condition, and from patient experience. We are hopeful that using these guidelines as a starting point, and with feedback from patients and physicians worldwide, we can evolve these guidelines over the next several years to make them increasingly cost-effective.

Upon HLRCC Diagnosis (At Any Age Greater Than 8)

- Full-body skin check by a dermatologist to note the location, number, and stage of skin bumps
- For all, MRI of the abdomen with thin cuts, looking for kidney tumors, noting number and size of any cysts or tumors seen
- Adults may be offered a CT scan as well as an MRI for their first appointment in order to have a baseline

scan for comparison with any later
scans

- For women starting at the age of 21,
  annual examinations by a gynecologist
  to enable screening for fibroids. You
  should inform the gynecologist that
  you have the HLRCC condition, of any
  family history of fibroids and stress the
  importance of looking for even small
  fibroids.

For Children at Risk Under 8

Children are "at risk" if they are not
genetically tested or if they are in the 3% of
families which have clear evidence of HLRCC
symptoms, but no DNA alteration can be found.

Annually from age 1

- Full body skin check by the
  pediatrician, noting any skin bumps.
  If present, refer to a dermatologist
  familiar with HLRCC

Annually beginning at age 8

- Full body skin check by the pediatrician
  noting any skin bumps. If present,
  refer to a dermatologist familiar with
  HLRCC

- MRI of the abdomen with thin cuts to
  check for any cysts or tumors of the
  kidneys. If present refer kidney issues
  to an urologist familiar with HLRCC.

Feedback—You Can Help Us Learn

Each time you do your annual check for any family member, would you please keep a log of the results? It is just as important for us to know that "all is well" as it is to hear that something was found. We are working to have a web-accessible, secure patient registry ready for your use within the next 1-2 years. Meanwhile, if you could please keep a paper notebook of this information, you will be able to add it when the online service is available. You will have an account and password to enter your information. Our goal is to analyze the medical information (without your personally identifying information) to determine at what ages the various issues are likely to emerge, and whether earlier intervention might be helpful. For example, there are new treatments for fibroids that might be used on smaller fibroids so that they never advance to the stage where hysterectomy is the only remaining option. See the fibroid section for treatment recommendations.

- Date
- Name of patient
- Date of birth
- Age of patient
- Skin check — please note what if anything was found. Include the location of any skin bumps, their color, number, and stage of development.
- Fibroid check (females only):
- Kidney check — note any cysts or tumors found. This information will be

spelled out in the written report from the scan. It would be a good idea for you to obtain a copy of this report and keep it in your notebook so you have it to refer back to in future.

- Any other health issues, whether or not they seem to be connected to HLRCC. Include blood pressure reading, any symptoms of kidney stones or infections, any irregularities in periods for females, any abnormalities noted in male scrotal exams, prostate, or epididymal cysts.

- Any treatments recommended?

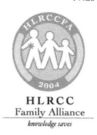

HLRCC
Family Alliance
knowledge saves

COMMONLY ASKED QUESTIONS

Who has HLRCC?

Males and females from birth, but most symptoms occur after puberty, which may begin as early as 8-9 years of age.

Should I get tested?

If one of your parents is positive for HLRCC, it is very important that you obtain a genetic test for yourself, either through the study at the US-NIH or through a genetic counselor. Remember — there is a 50% chance that you are negative. You will not be able to advocate for yourself and your family until you know for certain if you have HLRCC.

What is FH and why is it important to HLRCC?

FH stands for Fumarate Hydratase, an enzyme associated with the Krebs Cycle that naturally suppresses tumors. Individuals with HLRCC have a lower FH level than those without HLRCC.

Is there anything I can do about an FH enzyme deficiency?

At this point there is no enzyme replacement

for FH, but refer to our HLRCC Science document for the current research on enzyme replacement. http://hlrccinfo.org > Information > Science and Research, or http://www.hlrccinfo.org/science .

If I have HLRCC and have a child, should I have him/her tested?

This is a complex issue and there is no single answer or recommendation. We have written in this handbook a complete section on testing and screening as it is such an important issue.

What do I tell a child?

The level of information must be chosen to correspond to the child's age and their ability to understand. A genetic counselor is trained to help you in this and often is involved in an interview with the child. Obviously you don't want to scare the child, but hiding the simple facts by not discussing them may cause problems, especially with older children who can find out information by themselves and be more alarmed than is necessary. Children often have a surprising ability to cope with difficult news. Older children may be very angry with their parents if they feel that information was withheld from them when they were younger.

Is HLRCC a cancer?

Despite its name the majority of people with HLRCC never get kidney cancer and many people will go through life never knowing that they have HLRCC. Most of the tumors associated with HLRCC are not cancerous. The cutaneous leiomyoma (skin bumps) and uterine fibroids are problematic but benign. Some people (a minority) develop kidney cancer; but knowing about a genetic alteration and being able to screen for a cancer is a gift—an early warning system that most people do not have. It is best to find and treat kidney cancer before it has spread (called metastasis).

I am scared, how can I support myself and my family emotionally?

You have come to the right place. The HLRCC Family Alliance, found on the hlrccinfo.org site, has the information that you need. We also offer an e-mail address to send your questions to, a telephone number to discuss your concerns, and an online discussion at http://vhl.inspire.com in conjunction with other hereditary kidney cancers. We hope that you'll use these resources!

Further Reading—Internet Sites

Please refer to our HLRCC Science document for an extensive list of research articles. If you find an interesting article, please feel free to e-mail it to us as well!

The Science document can be found at http://hlrccinfo.org > Information > Science and Research, http://www.hlrccinfo.org/science .

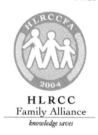

HLRCC
Family Alliance
knowledge saves

YOUR EMOTIONAL HEALTH

HLRCC can be an overwhelming diagnosis because of the word cancer. Although most HLRCC patients never get kidney cancer, dealing with the potential of developing it can be difficult. Others on this site may have learned of their HLRCC diagnosis AFTER developing kidney cancer and are currently undergoing medical treatment. No matter what stage you are experiencing, it is important to find emotional support to get you through this difficult time.

Some normal feelings after a diagnosis:

- Shock and Denial
- Fear and Worry
- Anger
- Sadness
- Acceptance and Coping

It can take one to two years after a diagnosis for life to return back to normal... and "normal" still means annual screening and always knowing that kidney cancer is a possibility. Having our children and family members tested can add to the stress of this diagnosis as well.

Being able to cope emotionally is essential for

staying healthy and fighting cancer. Stress is very powerful and too much stress can hurt the body's immune system. There are many things that you can do to help combat stress:

- Find time to exercise.Eat well and avoid tobacco, limit alcohol to 1-2 glasses per day and limit caffeine excesses.

- Get a good amount of sleep

- Surround yourself with positive people and family members/friends who will offer you emotional support.

- Find a support group to talk with about your feelings and fears.Attend individual, couple or family counseling.

- Become educated about HLRCC so you feel in control of your diagnosis. Purchase or download our handbook for detailed information.

- Find time to recharge your batteries. Depending on the type of person you are, either "Find quiet and alone time to clear your head" or "Find time to be with other people."

- Manage your stress, so that you feel more in control of your life. Use meditation, prayer, sports, walking, classical music, a bubble bath... to add something into your life that soothes you and helps you manage your stress level.

- Stay positive.

The HLRCC Family Alliance is a wonderful

support group of people and they can be found via the website www.hlrccinfo.org, and on Inspire, Facebook, and RareConnect as well. If you need a place to ask questions, find emotional support and talk about your own fears and feelings, please join us.

Patient and Medical Support

HLRCC Family Alliance Website

http://www.hlrccinfo.org

This is the home page for the HLRCC Family Alliance website and provides the central contact point

Inspire

http://vhl.inspire.com

The VHL Family Alliance Group in INSPIRE supports HLRCC and BHD as discussion topics. It provides private patient to patient message board support. It allows patients to talk with each other about their questions and concerns, while providing emotional support to one another. You can also write your own journal entries or start or add to discussion threads. There is privacy control. We strongly advise you to join and make friends.

You can look in on INSPIRE and then decide if you would like to join by creating your own user name and password. New topics are posted every day (there are many other topics discussed other than the specific medical issues of HLRCC) and it's a very easy way to connect with others who are impacted by HLRCC and related hereditary kidney cancer syndromes.

Facebook

http://www.facebook.com/groups/hlrcc/

This is a Facebook "Closed Group" HLRCC: Hereditary Leiomyomatosis and Renal Cell Cancer which means that posts can only be seen by members. Membership requests are controlled and accepted by the Group's administrators. This is an alternative or supplement to INSPIRE and appeals to those who have a Facebook account already. We strongly advise you to join and make friends. Members are finding this is a very easy way to communicate with each other.

RareConnect

http://hlrcc.rareconnect.org

This is a new support community for HLRCC in the organization RareConnect a partnership of Eurordis and NORD "Connecting Rare Disease Patients Globally". It is an alternative to INSPIRE, but has the advantage of providing language translation facilities. You can look in on RareConnect and then decide if you would like join by creating your own user name and password.

Kidney Cancer Facebook Group in UK

http://www.facebook.com/groups/195838270483807/

Connected to forum http://www.
kidneycancersupportnetwork.co.uk

Kidney Cancer Forums

These provide forums and message boards for
Kidney Cancer.

http://www.kidneycancer.me/

This is connected to the Kidney Cancer
Association see http://www.kidneycancer.org/

http://www.topix.com/forum/health/
kidney-cancer/

SMARTPATIENTS

https://www.smartpatients.com

Public launch April 2013 - This is a new, free
state-of-the art website. Smart Patients is an online
community for cancer patients and caregivers. The
community includes a clinical trial search engine
that presents trial data from ClinicalTrials.gov in a
patient-friendly format.

SmartPatients replaces the patient-to-patient
message board support KIDNEY-ONC and
PAPILLARY-RCC from the Association of Cancer
Online Resources (ACOR).

SmartPatients is an un-moderated discussion
lists for patients, family, friends, researchers and
physicians to discuss clinical and non-clinical
issues and advances pertaining to metastatic
kidney cancer, including renal cell cancer,
transitional cell carcinoma of the renal pelvis and
collecting duct carcinoma. This includes patient
experiences, psychosocial issues, new research,

clinical trials, alternative therapies and discussions of current treatment practices.

Other Sites

http://www.vitals.com/doctors

This is a free website for information about 700,000 practicing physicians in the United States.

http://www.apexmd.com

Free website for finding US Practitioners for named conditions. Search can be refined by area. Although HLRCC is not currently recognized, VHL is and many physicians cover both conditions. If you have searched by area, scroll down to the displayed information. Do not click on to any links as they will expand to the whole of the US. For example http://search.apexmd.com/search2.aspx?q=vhl&r=5 will show 9 urology physicians in Texas. Clicking on to the urology link will show all 1000 US physicians

http://www.caringbridge.org

Has free patient websites to help family and friends share information and support. This is particularly helpful for people who are currently in the hospital or undergoing longer treatments.

http://www.orpha.net/consor/

The portal for rare diseases and orphan drugs in Europe.

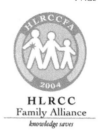

HLRCC
Family Alliance
knowledge saves

CLINICAL TRIALS

The list of clinical trials and studies is constantly changing and people are advised to seek out the latest information from your medical specialists or by contacting info@hlrccinfo.org . The following was current at the time of writing this document. Updates will be posted at http://www.hlrccinfo.org/trials .

The Natural History Study at the National Institutes of Health

The US-NIH, currently has a Natural History study for individuals who have been diagnosed with HLRCC or who have the clinical symptoms that might imply a possible diagnosis. The study is now seeing new people with HLRCC who have a kidney cyst or a solid tumor and also one new first person from a new family with HLRCC. Other people at risk in HLRCC families should be screened by their local medical centers.

If you have an interest in the US-NIH Study, contact:

Lindsay Middelton, RN, CGC
Urologic Oncology, National Cancer Inst.
Bldg. 10, CRC, Rm. 2W-5740

9000 Rockville Pike
Bethesda MD 20892
T: (301) 402-7911
F: (301) 435-9262
The US-NIH website: www.nih.gov

http://clinicaltrials.gov/ct/show/
NCT00050752?order=2

http://clinicalstudies.info.nih.gov/detail/
A_2003-C-0066.html

*"Genetic Study of Cancer Risk and Gene
Identification in Patients and Families With Hereditary
Leiomyomatosis and Renal Cell Cancer Syndrome"*

This study is currently recruiting participants
as of February 2013. http://clinicaltrials.gov/ct/
show/NCT00055627

Phase II Study of Bevacizumab and Erlotinib

http://clinicaltrialsfeeds.org/clinical-trials/show/NCT01130519

*"A Phase II Study of Bevacizumab and Erlotinib
in Subjects With Advanced Hereditary Leiomyomatosis
and Renal Cell Cancer (HLRCC) or Sporadic Papillary
Renal Cell Cancer"*

This clinical trial of bevacizumab (Avastin®
Genentech) and erlotinib (Tarceva® Genentech) is
currently recruiting patients with papillary kidney
cancer that has spread (metastasized) beyond
the kidneys. See also http://www.cancer.gov/
ncicancerbulletin/121410/page6

**http://www.aadmeetingnews.org/highlight.
aspx?id=2485&p=232**

W. Marston Linehan, M.D is reported as saying

*"As for HLRCC syndrome, NCI began focusing on this
familial kidney cancer syndrome in the 1980s. Researchers
learned that these patients develop a particularly aggressive
form of type 2 papillary kidney cancer. In addition to raised
and painful cutaneous leiomyomas, 90 percent of female
patients in these HLRCC syndrome families also develop
uterine fibroids."*

*"HLRCC is one of the most malignant types of kidney
cancer there is,"* Dr. Linehan said. *"It needs to be detected
because it can spread early and can be lethal."*

HLRCC syndrome is caused by an alteration
of the Krebs cycle enzyme, fumarate hydratase.
In studying this fumarate hydratase pathway
in HLRCC, NCI researchers learned that when
the fumarate hydratase gene in the cancer cell is
damaged, it alters its metabolism significantly,
becoming exceptionally dependent on glycolysis
and glucose uptake.

*"We have developed an approach to treatment that
involves using bevacizumab and erlotinib, therapeutic
agents that target the vulnerability of this fumarate
hydratase pathway in HLRCC patients with advanced
kidney cancer,"* Dr. Linehan said. *"This is currently an
ongoing clinical trial, and we are cautiously optimistic
about the early results."*

He also reported that blood tests are available
to assist clinicians in making a diagnosis by
detecting fumarate hydratase (FH) for HLRCC
syndrome and folliculin (FLCN) for BHD
syndrome.

*"In both of these hereditary cancer syndromes, it
is important for dermatologists and other clinicians*

*to understand the significance of fibrofolliculomas
and leiomyomas,"* Dr. Linehan said. *"These patients
need to be evaluated for the possible presence of kidney
cancer when they present with these dermatologic
findings."*

Listen to W. Marston Linehan, M.D

http://www.hlrccinfo.org/audio/Linehan.
mp3

**Editor's Note: Additional drugs will
be forthcoming that will target the FH
pathway.   Stay tuned for more news.**

Treatment of Cutaneous Leiomyomas with Botulinum Toxin

http://clinicalstudies.info.nih.gov/cgi/detail.
cgi?A_2009-C-0072.html

http://bethesdatrials.cancer.gov/clinical-research/
cts.aspx?ProtocolID=NCI-09-C-0072

"Randomized Pilot Study for the Treatment of
Cutaneous Leiomyomas with Botulinum Toxin"

This study is currently recruiting participants.

Intravenous Recombinant Human IL-15

http://www.clinicaltrials.gov/ct2/show/
NCT01021059

"A Phase I Study of Intravenous Recombinant
Human IL-15 in Adults With Refractory Metastatic
Malignant Melanoma and Metastatic Renal Cell
Cancer"

This study is currently recruiting participants.

Extensive List of Relevant Research Articles

Please refer to our separate "HLRCC Science" document (http://www.hlrccinfo.org/science).

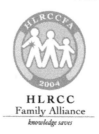

HLRCC
Family Alliance
knowledge saves

BACKGROUND OF THE TERM
HLRCC

Since the 1950s some benign skin lumps were known to be inherited in some families and the cells have a distinctive appearance under a microscope see *Hereditary Multiple Leiomyoma of The Skin,* Warner et al. 1958, PMID: PMC1931875

Full text:

http://www.ncbi.nlm.nih.gov/pmc/articles/PMC1931875/pdf/ajhg00572-0055.pdf

However the term "myoma" was defined a hundred years before by Virchow in 1854.

The lumps were termed "cutaneous leiomyomas", "cutaneous piloleiomyomas" or "cutaneous pilar leiomyomas." These are benign smooth muscle tumors arising from the arrectores pilorum (singular: arrector pili) muscles associated with the hair follicles of the skin.

Cutaneous leiomyomas are made up of a poorly circumscribed proliferation of haphazardly arranged smooth muscle fibers located in the dermis that appear to infiltrate the surrounding tissue and may extend into the subcutis.

The term "multiple cutaneous leiomyoma"

(MCL) was used when several lumps were
present. They occur in clusters or singly on arms,
legs, and trunk and sometimes on the face. There
is a classification of Type 1 for solitary and Type 2
for multiple in cluster patterns. It was then noted
by W.B. Reed *et al.* in a published paper in 1973
that females with this condition also invariably
had uterine leiomyomas (fibroids).

The term Reed's Syndrome or "multiple
cutaneous and uterine leiomyomas" (MCUL) was
then used to describe this condition. MCL and
MCUL are defined in the definition of HLRCC in
the Online Mendelian Inheritance in Man (OMIM):
http://www.ncbi.nlm.nih.gov/omim/150800

It was nearly 30 years later in 2001 that
V. Launonen *et al.* published a paper linking
malignant kidney cancer to the syndrome. This
was a major advance from a relatively benign
condition to a much more serious possibility
of malignant cancer and the term "hereditary
leiomyomatosis and renal cell cancer" (HLRCC)
was used to describe the condition when kidney
cancer was present. HLRCC is defined in MIM ID
#605839

http://www.ncbi.nlm.nih.gov/omim/605839

In 2002 I.P. Tomlinson *et al.* identified
alterations in the FH gene as being responsible.

To date there are over a 100 different FH
gene alterations described in a genetic database.
http://www.biomedcentral.com/1471-2350/9/20

Unfortunately all these terms are in use
to relate to the one condition — MCL, MCUL,

MCUL1, Reed's or Reed Syndrome, HLRCC, LRCC, Fumarate Hydratase (FH) Gene Alteration and Fumarase. This makes searching for information on the Internet very difficult. The acronym HLRCC is not always present to help the search. Also do not be confused by a completely unrelated condition called Familial hypercholesterolemia (abbreviated FH or Fh).

There is further opportunity for misunderstanding in that the Fumarate Hydratase (FH) Gene Alteration is responsible for two distinct conditions. (1) HLRCC and (2) Fumarase Deficiency.

This Handbook is mainly concerned with **hereditary leiomyomatosis and renal cell cancer** – caused by single alterations in the FH gene. There is a separate section in this book on Fumarase Deficiency.

Over 100 alterations in the FH gene that cause hereditary leiomyomatosis and renal cell cancer (HLRCC) have now been reported. Most of these alterations replace one amino acid with another amino acid in the fumarase enzyme.

People with HLRCC are born with one altered copy of the FH gene in each cell. The second copy of the FH gene in certain cells may also acquire alterations as a result of environmental factors such as ultraviolet radiation from the sun or a mistake that occurs as DNA copies itself during cell division. These changes are called somatic mutations and are not inherited.

FH gene alterations interfere with the enzyme's role in the citric acid cycle, resulting in a buildup of fumarate. Researchers believe that the excess fumarate may interfere with the oxygen level detection system in the cell. Stabilization of hypoxia inducible factor (HIF) due to pseudohypoxia (false indication of low oxygen even when oxygen is plentiful) in cells with two altered copies of the FH gene may encourage tumor formation and result in the tendency to develop leiomyomas and renal cell cancer."

MIM ID *136850 describes the FH gene in http://www.ncbi.nlm.nih.gov/omim/136850

FUMARASE DEFICIENCY

Happens when **BOTH** parents have an FH alteration

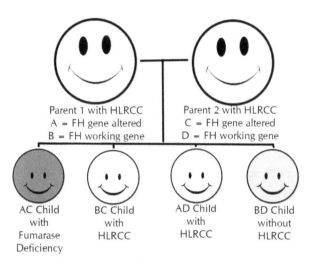

Figure 10: Inheritance of Fumarase Deficiency, a recessive characteristic. From Genetics Home Reference: http://ghr.nlm.nih.gov/gene/FH

Each child gets one copy of the FH gene from each parent.

In this way, there are four possible arrangements of these four genes. Each arrangement has a 25% chance. So there is a 50% chance of having HLRCC and a 25% chance of having fumarase deficiency and a 25% of not having either condition.

As shown in Figure 9, there is a 25% chance of developing Fumarase Deficiency based on both parents having a FH alteration. Fumarase Deficiency is a Autosomal Recessive condition as it requires both genes to have alterations (though not necessarily the same alteration).

Fumarase deficiency is caused by alterations in the FH gene usually from both parents. It is also known by the name of fumaric aciduria.

Approximately 17 FH gene alterations that cause fumarase deficiency have been reported. However many (if not all) FH gene alterations combinations probably have the potential to cause this condition, but are not seen because they would be incompatible with fetal life. Fumarase deficiency occurs in individuals who inherit two altered copies of the FH gene in each cell. (This is different from HLRCC, in which individuals have one altered copy and one normal copy of FH in each cell). In fumarase deficiency, most of these alterations replace one protein building block (amino acid) with another amino acid in the fumarase enzyme. These changes disrupt the ability of the enzyme to help convert fumarate to malate, interfering with the function of this reaction in the citric acid cycle. Impairment of the process that generates energy for cells is particularly harmful to cells in the developing brain, and this impairment results in the signs and symptoms of fumarase deficiency (also known as fumaricaciduria). This is defined in MIM ID #606812 http://www.ncbi.nlm.nih.gov/omim/606812 . Fumarase deficiency has had widespread publicity because of its polygamy connections see http://www.childbrides.org/taxes_PNT_forbidden_fruit.html

However there are several cases where the parents are unrelated to each other.

Symptoms and Diagnosis

The condition has considerable variation from relatively mild symptoms to very severe leading to an early death. The new born baby has brain defects leading to seizures and doesn't develop normally. There may be distinctive facial appearance. This link http://rarediseases.info.nih.gov/GARD/Condition/6476/QnA/37149/Fumarase_deficiency.aspx provides a more comprehensive description. A high level of fumaric acid level in the urine is a key indicator. MRI scans of the brain can be used to see the extent of malformation. A genetic test to determine the FH gene alterations is the definitive test. The parents would also be tested for FH gene alteration as they would normally each have the HLRCC condition.

Treatment and Management

There is no cure for fumarase deficiency and treatment is attending to the conditions symptomatically to prevent further harm, as in the case of seizures. Depending on severity suitable diets may help with feeding difficulties and a wheelchair to provide physical support may be useful.

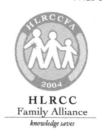

HLRCC
Family Alliance
knowledge saves

HOW DO CHANGES IN DNA CAUSE CHANGES IN FUMARASE?

If your genetic test results show that you have an alteration in your fumarase gene, you may have questions about what the letters, numbers, and symbols that describe the alteration mean. You may also wonder how changes in the DNA of your fumarase gene interfere with the making of fumarase in your cells.

**Figure 11: Diagram of the FH Gene
with Coding DNA Nucleotide Numbers
(not to scale)**

intron # (length)	1 (2274)		2 (3468)	3 (1459)	4 (3181)		5 (2434)	6 (1757)	7 (1471)	8 (1852)	9 (2466)	

exon #	1	2		3	4		5	6	7	8	9	10
start	-63*	133		268	379		556	739	905	1109	1237	1391
end	132	267		378	555		738	904	1108	1236	1390	

* negative numbered nucleotides are "upstream" of the RNA transcription start point and contain transcription promoter sequences. Information from LOVD TCA Cycle Gene Mutation Database.

Krebs Cycle

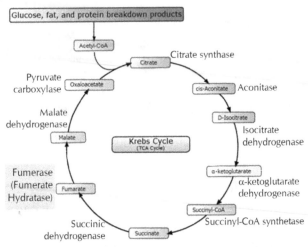

Figure 12: The Krebs Cycle

The Krebs Cycle was discovered by Hans A. Krebs. It takes place in the innermost space of the mitochondria and requires the presence of oxygen. Together with the electron transport chain, it produces most of the cells' energy.

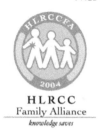

HLRCC
Family Alliance
knowledge saves

GLOSSARY:
DEFINITIONS OF COMMONLY USED HLRCC TERMS

Assay – Used to measure the quantity of fumarase enzyme in a sample of skin cells.

Autosomal – when the gene defect is located on one of the 22 regular chromosomes and not on a sex chromosome (X or Y). The result is that males and females may have the condition, in approximately equal numbers.

Citric Acid Cycle – see Krebs Cycle.

CT Scan – Computed Tomography also known as CAT (Computerized Axial Tomography) uses a computer to combine many x-ray images to generate cross-sectional views and 3-dimensional images of internal organs and structures of the body.

Cutaneous – Pertaining to the skin – not only the skin surface, but also in the skin layers.

Dominant – a gene is dominant when it is only necessary to have one altered copy of the gene in order to have the condition. Consequently, if the gene is autosomal (on a chromosome other than the X or Y chromosome), there is a 50% chance of a child inheriting the condition.

FH — Fumarate Hydratase, the enzyme encoded by the gene associated with HLRCC

Fibroid — is a benign (non-cancerous) tumor that originates from the smooth muscle layer of the uterus and its connective tissue. It is a uterine leiomyoma.

Fumarase — (or fumarate hydratase) is an enzyme that catalyzes the reversible hydration/dehydration of Fumarate to S-malate in the Krebs Cycle.

Fumarate — This chemical is formed during the basic cell energy cycle known as the Citric Acid Cycle or Krebs Cycle.

Genotype – This is the specific genetic information of the cells in your body.

HLRCC — Hereditary Leiomyomatosis and Renal Cell Cancer.

Hereditary — passed from one generation to the next.

Krebs Cycle — is a series of chemical reactions which is used by all aerobic living organisms to generate energy through the oxidization of acetate derived from carbohydrates, fats and proteins into carbon dioxide and water.

Leiomyoma — an abnormal growth of smooth muscle tissue. In HLRCC there are cutaneous and uterine leiomyoma.

Leiomyomata — the correct Latin plural form of leiomyoma. However most articles now use leiomyomas instead.

Leiomyomatosis—means the occurrence of leiomyomas in the body.

LOH—Loss of Heterozygosity—HLRCC tumors are found to have no fumarase activity, which is termed Loss of Heterozygosity (LOH) for FH. The two alleles of the FH gene were different (one altered) but now they are both altered. This represents the "second hit" to FH gene function in this one cell, the loss of the normal function of the second copy of the FH gene through somatic alteration.

Metastasize—when cancerous cells break off from the primary tumor and travel to other parts of the body and start new secondary tumors.

MRI Scan—Magnetic resonance imaging, a type of scan that uses no ionizing radiation. It provides good contrast between the different soft tissues of the body. Gadolinium contrast is used to enhance the 3d-image.

PET/CT Scan—Positron Emission Tomography (PET) combined with an x-ray Computed Tomography (CT) is used to trace glucose metabolism (using fluorodeoxyglucose, FDG). High uptake is seen in HLRCC tumors. http://www.radiologyinfo.org/en/info. cfm?pg=pet .

Phenotype—These are the actual observed symptoms that you have which researchers try to match to your genetic alteration – see *Genotype*.

Piloleiomyoma—the full name of the benign skin lump, sometimes preceded by the word "cutaneous" or shortened to just "leiomyoma"

Primary Tumor — a tumor which has developed in its original place, grown from a single cell.

Progress — to continue to get worse, a term used for cancer which has worsened, such as increased tumor size or cancer spread.

Recessive — a gene is recessive when it is necessary to have two altered copies of the gene in order to have the condition (though not necessarily the same alteration).

Remission — used in conjunction with the words "*complete*" and "*partial*". Complete remission is no sign of any remaining cancer. Partial remission is an improvement, tumor shrinkage or less activity etc.

Clear cell Renal Cell Carcinoma (RCC) — is the most common type of kidney cancer in adults (carcinoma = a type of cancer).

RCC Classification — there are many forms of RCC, including Clear Cell (most common), Papillary I and II, Clear Cell Tubulopapillary, Chromophobe, Oncocytic, Collecting Duct and Non-classified. Classification of the cell type is made by a pathologist trained in the types of renal cancer.

Scan Types — There are several different types of scan — See entries for MRI, CT, PET/CT, Ultrasound, and Bone.

TCA — tricarboxylic acid cycle see Krebs Cycle.

Ultrasound Scan — An ultrasound scan is a painless test that uses sound waves to create images of organs and structures inside your body.

It can be used on kidneys, but there is a risk that not all tumors will be detected. In HLRCC it can be useful to track fibroids in the uterus.

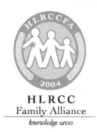

HLRCC
Family Alliance
knowledge saves

HANDOUTS FOR PRINTING

On the following pages is a separate small document which can be modified for your own use. You might also consider printing our Quick Facts and HLRCC Brochure which can be obtained from our website www.hlrccinfo.org

Sample Family Letter (to send to relatives of someone recently diagnosed with HLRCC)

To Members of the _____ Family,

I hope this letter finds all of you happy and in good health. My main reason for writing this is to inform my relatives of a hereditary medical condition that I have been diagnosed with. The condition is extremely rare in the general population, but it runs in families. Since I have it, this means that others in the family are at risks up to 50%. It is called Hereditary Leiomyomatosis and Renal Cell Cancer (HLRCC). The kidney cancer component of this disease can be fatal if not treated in time.

I am hoping that you will act on this information since this is a hereditary condition. We all have a risk as high as 50% of having the gene alteration. If we have it, our children have a 50% chance of having it (and so on). Consequently, some members of a particular branch of the family may have members with the condition while others are free of it. Having a genetic test is the best way to be diagnosed with the condition. Even if you decide not to be genetically tested I encourage you to seek screening advice, actions you can take to watch for signs of trouble.

People with this condition are susceptible to the development of the following:

- **Uterine Fibroids in females**, often early onset, multiple, large and symptomatic, usually detected in the 20's and 30's, may impact the ability to have children, and often lead to hysterectomy.
- **Skin Leiomyomas** (non-cancerous

growth) of the skin, usually on the stomach, back, arms and legs, can be isolated or clustered lesions or can be disseminated (segmental), sometimes painful or may not hurt, and typically onset is in 30's but have been seen in children. They usually appear as small firm, pink raised growths (sometimes white) or bumps in clusters and are difficult to diagnose yourself: http://www.dermnet.com/Leiomyomata/photos/1

- **Kidney Cancer** — individual risk is not completely known at this time, but a high percentage of adults with this condition have been found to have kidney tumors. The average age of symptomatic kidney cancer is 44, but we think that survival is better when tumors are found before symptoms occur. Even children have been diagnosed with this type of kidney cancer

- Those with HLRCC need to be screened annually for kidney tumors, preferably by a thin sliced MRI with contrast. Even small tumors have been known to metastasize (spread) so annual screening is the very best way to catch tumors as early as possible.

The HLRCC Family Alliance is a strong organization that can help address your questions and concerns. Go to **http://www.hlrccinfo.org** to access a detailed handbook and to join the support group. You can also find information about a large on-going study at the National Institutes of Health (US-NIH) that you may be able to participate in should you test positive for HLRCC.

Please call me at _____ to discuss this letter further.   You can also call their Hotline number:

> 1-800-767-4845 extension 709 (toll-free)
>
> or +1-617-277-5667 extension 709
>
> E-mail: info@hlrccinfo.org

or write to:

> HLRCC Family Alliance c/o VHLFA,
>
> 2001 Beacon Street,
>
> Suite 208, Boston,
>
> MA 02135
>
> USA

Love to you all.

HLRCC FAMILY ALLIANCE

c/o VHL Family Alliance
2001 Beacon Street, Suite 208,
Boston, MA 02135-7787 USA
Tel: +1 617-277-5667 Ext 709,
Fax: +1-858-712-8712
+1 800 767-4845 Ext 709,
toll-free from US, Canada, Mexico
E-mail: info@hlrccinfo.org
www.hlrccinfo.org

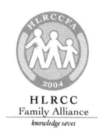

HLRCC
Family Alliance
knowledge saves

CPSIA information can be obtained
at www.ICGtesting.com
Printed in the USA
LVHW081943080522
718111LV00028BA/472